Fit Pregnancy

Optimal Prenatal Nutrition and Exercise

Table of Contents

Chapter 1. Introduction

In this Special Report, we explore the electric environment of 'Fit Pregnancy,' where the unmatched beauty of motherhood meets optimal prenatal nutrition and exercise routines. It's not about complex statistics or scientific jargon—rather we delve into accessible, practical steps to ensure both you and your unborn child thrive during this miraculous journey. Bursting with expert-recommended diet advice, exhilarating workouts, and inspirational real-life stories, this guide can become your trusted companion during pregnancy. Let's create the healthiest possible start for your little one together—and guess what? You don't need to be a fitness guru or a nutritionist to get it right. Come, embark on this empowering journey—nurture your body and nourish your baby, growing stronger side by side! Brace yourself, because after reading this report, embracing a fit pregnancy will be as natural as your baby's first kick.

Chapter 2. Understanding the Dynamics of a Fit Pregnancy

The journey through pregnancy is unique and beautiful; a period filled with anticipation, hope, and a world of emotions. The nine months of pregnancy can be joyous, bewildering, and sometimes challenging. As an expectant parent, you may have numerous questions about how to ensure the health and fitness of both yourself and your growing baby. This chapter will guide you through the dynamics of maintaining a 'fit' pregnancy, from nutrition to exercise and beyond. It aims to address your queries, dispel myths, and arm you with the effective tools to ensure a healthy, vibrant pregnancy.

2.1. A Glimpse into Prenatal Nutrition

The famous adage, 'eating for two,' is often misinterpreted as a license to eat twice as much. In reality, optimal prenatal nutrition focuses on the quality of food intake rather than the quantity. Your diet should be a balance of proteins, carbohydrates, healthy fats, vitamins, and minerals.

Your baby's growth depends on your nutrition, therefore, ensuring you consume a healthy diet is important. High-quality proteins support the growth of fetal tissue, including the brain. Whole grains provide necessary energy, fiber, and iron. Fruits and vegetables, filled with vitamins and antioxidants, promote the overall development of the unborn child.

Consider these food groups in your daily meal plan: - Dairy: High in calcium and protein, dairy products support your baby's bone development. Include milk, cheese, and yoghurt in your diet. - Proteins: Lean meats, eggs, legumes, and nuts are good protein sources. - Carbohydrates: Opt for whole grains over refined. They provide energy and help you feel full. - Fruits and vegetables: These provide vitamins, fiber, and are often low in calories.

Try to consume a variety of foods to cover every nutrient your body and baby requires. Consider also prenatal vitamins to fill any nutritional gaps, particularly for nutrients like folic acid and iron. Consult your doctor before starting any dietary supplements.

2.2. Deciphering Exercise During Pregnancy

Exercise during pregnancy carries innumerable benefits, such as enhanced mood, decreased pregnancy discomfort, and preparation for labor and birth. But where do you begin?

First, it's imperative to consult with your healthcare provider before starting or continuing any exercise routine during pregnancy. Once you get the green signal, go ahead gradually, working your way up from low impact to moderate intensity exercises.

Common exercises suitable for pregnant women include: - Walking: This is a safe activity to initiate and it can be carried right through the entire pregnancy. - Prenatal yoga or Pilates: Helps improve flexibility, balance, and muscle tone. - Swimming: This provides a whole-body workout, is gentle on the joints, and can alleviate swelling and discomfort.

Remember, the goal is not to set new fitness records, but to maintain a healthy level of physical activity.

2.3. Understanding the Impact on Mental Health

Pregnancy is a time of psychological and physiological changes. Hormonal shifts can lead to mood swings, anxiety, or melancholy. Regular exercise and a balanced diet have proven benefits for mental health. Yoga, in particular, with its emphasis on breathing and mindfulness, can help to tame stress and enhance mood.

2.4. Dispelling Pregnancy Fitness Myths

Misinformation surrounding pregnancy fitness can be confusing. Always ask your healthcare provider if you're unsure.

Myth 1: "Exercise can harm the baby." Fact: Regular, moderate-intensity exercise is not only safe, but also beneficial for most pregnant women.

Myth 2: "You must eat twice as much during pregnancy." Fact: Quality trumps quantity. Aim for a nutrient-rich diet, not extra portions.

Knowing the dynamics of prenatal nutrition, exercise, and mental wellness ensures a fit, healthy pregnancy. As individual as the journey is, there's a wealth of science-backed advice available to guide each step. Above all, listen to your body, remain active, and nourish both yourself and your little one towards a memorable journey of motherhood.

Chapter 3. Preserving Health: The Role of Nutrition Before Pregnancy

Emphasizing the indispensable role of nutrition before conception, it's crucial to understand that the health and diet practices adopted during this time serve as the bedrock of a fit pregnancy. An optimal diet ensures a fertile terrain, ready for the miraculous journey of development and growth that lies ahead.

3.1. The Power of Balanced Meals

In order to provide rich soil for the growth of a new life, your body should be brimming with essential nutrients. Begin by ensuring your meals are balanced, encompassing all realms of nutrients: proteins, carbohydrates, healthy fats, vitamins, and minerals.

Under the umbrella of proteins are building blocks, also referred to as amino acids. Key in every cell's development, proteins are crucial for both the mother's and the baby's health. Lean meats, dairy, legumes, and seeds are excellent sources.

Carbohydrates provide the body with energy. Opt for complex carbohydrates—like whole grains, fruits, and vegetables—that are digested slower, providing a steady supply of energy, while negating sudden blood sugar spikes.

Adopt a 'rainbow plate' strategy: incorporating an array of fruits and vegetables in your diet—each color signifies a particular group of nutrients—to ensure you are absorbing a wide range of vitamins and minerals.

Healthy fats provide fuel for the body and aid in brain development.

Avocado, oily fish, nuts, and seeds should be included as they are teeming with Omega-3 and Omega-6 fatty acids.

3.2. Prioritize Folic Acid

Understand that folic acid, or folate, is vital pre-pregnancy and in the early stages of gestation as it significantly reduces the risk of serious neural tube defects. Amplify your intake of folic acid by integrating dark leafy greens, legumes, citrus fruits, and fortified cereals into your diet.

3.3. Maintain a Healthy Weight

Strive to attain a balanced weight before pregnancy according to the Body Mass Index (BMI). If you're overweight or underweight, you increase the risks of gestational diabetes, hypertension, birth complications, and cardiovascular issues. Regular exercise along with an appropriate diet are key.

3.4. Nutrient-Rich Diet: Addressing Potential Shortfalls

Even with a balanced diet, you may not be acquiring the full range of nutrients essential for a successful pregnancy and healthy baby. Calcium, Iron, and Vitamin D are usually deficient in most women. Consider upping intake of foods rich in these nutrients, or discuss a suitable supplement regimen with your healthcare provider.

3.5. Hydrate, Hydrate, Hydrate

Water is responsible for the delivery of necessary nutrients to cells, aiding in digestion and absorption of these nutrients into your blood. Furthermore, hydration aids in the prevention of urinary tract infections and constipation, which are common during pregnancy.

3.6. Limit Intake of Caffeine and Completely Avoid Alcohol

While experts recommend limiting the consumption of caffeinated drinks, alcohol must be entirely avoided during pregnancy and even before conception, as it can lead to birth defects and developmental issues.

3.7. Embracing an Active Lifestyle

Ensuring a healthy diet is paired with an active lifestyle will hugely benefit you in the upcoming journey. Regular exercise, whether it is light walking, swimming or yoga, boosts overall health, reduces pregnancy-related complications, and helps you manage your weight.

3.8. The Role of a Nutritionist

It may be beneficial to consult a nutritionist or dietitian before you conceive. They could design a tailored plan that ensures all nutrient minimums are met and dispel any myths surrounding pre-pregnancy diets.

Wholesome and well-rounded nutrition is paramount to creating a nurturing habitat for your little one. A balanced diet, teeming with a variety of nutrients, primes your body for the upcoming journey of pregnancy. Not only does it help to maintain optimal health for you, but it also provides the life-supporting supplements needed for baby's healthy development. By intelligently combining your meals, you guarantee that you're best suited for the journey ahead. Rest assured, with nutrition at the heart of your strategy, building a stronger, healthier motherhood is well within reach.

Remember to balance your routine with regular light exercise, adequate rest, staying well-hydrated, and ensuring regular health screenings. Taking care of yourself is the first step towards taking care of your unborn child. As you embark on this journey, remember the importance of good nutrition: fueling your body, nurturing your baby, and sculpting a healthy future for both of you.

Chapter 4. Building Blocks of Prenatal Nutrition: Micros to Macros

The womb is nature's most miraculous incubator, a warm and secure environment specifically designed to cultivate and nurture life. Much like a flower requires the right balance of sunshine, water, and nutrients for optimal growth, your unborn child requires a fine-tuned balance of micro and macro nutrients from you, the expectant mother, to develop fully and healthily. Although pregnancy cravings might push you towards sugar-loaded treats, remember: the sweets might momentarily satisfy your sweet tooth, but they do very little to promote your baby's growth and development.

4.1. Understanding Macronutrients

Macronutrients are nutrients that our bodies require in larger amounts for energy production, muscle function, hormone synthesis, and body repair. They include proteins, carbohydrates, and fats.

Protein is the superstar macronutrient during pregnancy, playing paramount roles like repairing cells, building muscles, producing hormones, and contributing to your baby's growth — literally building every cell of your newborn baby's body.

Carbohydrates provide the energy needed to carry out daily functions, including the energy to power your growing baby's brain. Choose complex carbohydrates—like whole grains, fruits, and vegetables—for slow-releasing energy, dietary fiber, and essential vitamins and minerals.

Fats absorb some essential vitamins and produce vital fatty acids. While it's important to get enough 'good fats' from sources like avocados, nuts, seeds, and fatty fish for the development of your baby's brain and cells, be mindful to limit 'bad fats,' including trans-fats and saturated fats.

4.2. Embracing Micronutrients

Micronutrients, though required by our bodies in smaller amounts, are vital to health and development. These include vitamins and minerals that serve a variety of crucial roles, from boosting immune function to assisting in cellular functions like energy production and DNA synthesis.

Among the most crucial micronutrients during pregnancy is iron, which helps to carry oxygen in the blood — to both your body and your baby's. Folate is another pregnancy superstar, helping prevent neural tube defects. Calcium aids in the formation of your baby's bones and teeth, while iodine supports proper brain and nervous system development.

4.3. Tailoring Your Prenatal Nutrition

Just because you're 'eating for two' doesn't mean you should double your food portions. Instead, shift your focus on making every mouthful nutrient-dense. Capitalize on the power of a balanced diet, full of fresh fruits, vegetables, whole grains, lean proteins, and healthy fats.

While it's feasible to get most nutrients from your diet, prenatal vitamins can act as 'nutrient insurance' to cover any gaps. A high-quality prenatal supplement should comprise the vital nutrients that your baby needs, including folic acid, iron, calcium, Vitamin D, DHA, and iodine.

However, supplements aren't a substitute for a wholesome diet.

Make sure they are part of a broader healthful eating plan.

4.4. Navigating Pregnancy Pains with Nutrition

Many common pregnancy ailments can be alleviated—or even prevented—through a well-nourished diet. For instance, morning sickness is less intense when you're well-hydrated and your stomach is never empty, so try to take small, frequent meals and sip on water throughout the day. Heartburn, a common issue in later pregnancy, can be lessened by eating smaller, more frequent meals, avoiding foods and drinks that trigger heartburn, and not lying down soon after eating.

In case of gestational diabetes, balancing carbohydrates with proteins and fats and opting for high-fiber foods can help maintain blood sugar levels. For pregnancy-induced hypertension or preeclampsia, while it's vital to follow your healthcare provider's advice, a diet with ample fruits and vegetables, lean proteins, whole grains, and restricted salt may be beneficial.

4.5. Hydration: The Forgotten Nutrient

Water is a silent hero in prenatal nutrition. It plays critical roles in digestion, nutrient absorption, and transportation. Hydration is doubly important during pregnancy to support the increased blood volume and amniotic fluid.

Finally, every pregnancy is unique. Pay due attention to your body's responses, and adjust your dietary plan as necessary. Prenatal nutrition isn't a one-size-fits-all solution. You might need to experiment and adapt your approach depending on what your body and baby need, in consultation with your healthcare provider.

Bringing life into the world is no minor feat—it is a journey of love and patience, of growth and resilience. These building blocks of prenatal nutrition are a roadmap designed to guide you and your little one in this wonderful journey, empowering you to make each meal you consume work for both you and your growing baby. By meeting each day of your pregnancy with self-love and optimal nutrition, you create the best possible environment for your baby—one meal, one bite, and one breath at a time.

Chapter 5. Movement Matters: The Science of Prenatal Exercise

The fundamental joy of feeling your baby grow inside you is enhanced by the incredible physiological and psychological benefits made possible through a well-rounded prenatal exercise routine. You're not just supporting your body as it navigates these transformative nine months, but also engineering an optimum physical environment for your developing child.

5.1. The Anatomy of Prenatal Exercise

Understanding the underlying science of prenatal exercise begins with recognizing the profound changes that occur in your body. Your heart grows physically larger to support the increased blood volume—around 40-50% higher than pre-pregnancy rates. This adaptational marvel allows adequate oxygen and nutrients to reach both the mother and the developing fetus.

When you exercise, this increased blood volume is maximized further. This heightened circulation considerably boosts the delivery of oxygen and nourishment to your baby and helps eliminate waste products more efficiently. Increased blood flow also supports essential functions like digestion, improving your ability to absorb nutrients from your diet, which in turn, positively influences fetal growth and development.

5.2. To Kegel or Not to Kegel

The changes brought about by pregnancy aren't just on a giant, whole-body scale. There's one specific muscle group—the pelvic floor—that has a central role. These are the muscles that provide support to the uterus, bladder, and bowels.

Pelvic floor exercises, commonly known as Kegel exercises, are critical in maintaining the strength and tone of these muscles. The increased weight exerted by a growing uterus can strain and weaken your pelvic floor, leading to issues such as incontinence during and after pregnancy. Regular Kegel exercises can prevent these problems and also help in labor and delivery by improving your ability to push effectively.

Try visualizing your pelvic floor muscles as a hammock, extending from your pubic bone at the front to the base of your spine at the back. To perform a Kegel, squeeze the muscles as if you are trying to halt urination in midstream. Hold the squeeze for 10 seconds, then release gradually.

5.3. Aerobics and Cardiovascular Health

Aerobic exercise is another essential ingredient of a comprehensive prenatal fitness plan. It not only strengthens your heart and lungs but also helps you manage your weight, improves your mood, and promotes better sleep.

Exercise recommendations vary depending on your pre-pregnancy fitness levels. However, a common point of agreement among experts is that most pregnant women should aim for at least 150 minutes of moderate-intensity exercise each week.

Walking and swimming are excellent modes of low-impact aerobic exercise. They bear the weight of your changing body, reduce the risk of joint injuries, and can be continued right up to delivery. Alternatively, pre-natal aerobics classes or dance-based workouts like Zumba can offer fun and social ways to stay fit.

5.4. Strength Training: Supporting Your Changing Body

Pregnancy comes along with its own set of physical challenges. As your belly grows, there's an increased load placed on your back and upper body. This shift can affect your posture and cause plenty of discomforts if not supported by a strong musculature.

Strength training can help. When performed under right guidance, these exercises can strengthen your back, arms, shoulders, and legs, alleviating pregnancy discomforts. Bodyweight exercises like wall push-ups, chair squats, or lunges can be beneficial. Superwomen, where you alternate lifting your right arm and left leg and then swapping to the opposite pairs, is a superb exercise to strengthen your lower back.

While strength training, remember to avoid holding your breath or any high-intensity moves. Always listen to your body and avoid workout positions where you're lying flat on your back, which can restrict blood flow to your baby.

5.5. Yoga: Flexibility and Relaxation

Yoga isn't just about staying limber. It can profoundly calm your mind, relieve stress, and prepare your body for the process of labour. Research indicates that practicing prenatal yoga can even reduce the risk of preterm labor and intrauterine growth restriction—a condition that slows a baby's growth.

Look for yoga classes specifically designed for expectant mothers.

These classes offer poses that are safe and beneficial during different stages of pregnancy, and they avoid postures that can strain or overstretch your muscles.

5.6. When Exercise Might Not Be Safe

Despite myriad benefits that prenatal exercise boasts of, there are a few exceptions where it's best to rest or seek medical advice. If you experience persistent shortness of breath, dizziness, chest pain, or fluid leakage, it's best to stop exercising and talk to your healthcare provider. Also, if you have a chronic condition like heart disease, asthma, or diabetes, you should also consult with your doctor before beginning or continuing a workout regimen.

Remember, pregnancy isn't a time to push athletic boundaries. Instead, it's an opportunity to nurture your body with gentle, supportive exercises that prepare you for the journey ahead—an empowering journey of motherhood.

After all, it's not just about exercising for two—it's about paving the way for a healthy, radiant life for your little one. As you lace up your walking shoes or slip on your yoga mat, remember each step, each stretch isn't just for you. It's for the baby who will soon become the best part of your lives. Fitness isn't an end goal—it's the journey. A journey of love, care, health, and togetherness.

To sum up, the science of prenatal exercise is an encompassing one, extending beyond the realms of merely staying active. It embraces your changing body, it cherishes the growing life within, it prepares you for the beautiful journey forthcoming. With each pulse, each perspiration bead, let the marvel of motherhood dawn upon you, enriching both your life and the little one waiting to see the world.

Chapter 6. Designing Your Ideal Prenatal Workout Routine

As you embark on this journey towards motherhood, now is the best time to design your perfect prenatal workout routine. Not only does exercising help keep you fit, but it also prepares your body for the physical demands of pregnancy and childbirth. Here's your complete guide to creating a program that nurtures your body while making room for the new life inside.

6.1. Getting Started: Speak to Your Doctor

Before you start any new workout regimen, the first step is to consult your doctor or midwife. Pregnancy affects everyone differently, and what might be safe for one person might not be safe for another. Your healthy pregnancy workout plan should be personalized to you, considering your fitness level, overall health, and any potential complications. Also, if you've been participating in a sport or exercise routine before pregnancy, your practitioner will guide you on how to modify it accordingly.

6.2. Understand Your Body's Changes

Understanding the changes your body undergoes during pregnancy will play a crucial role in designing your ideal prenatal workout routine. When pregnant, your body produces a hormone called relaxin that loosens your joints and ligaments to prepare for childbirth. While this eases delivery, it can also increase your risk of injury during strenuous or high-impact workouts. Additionally, your increased blood volume and shifting center of gravity could affect your balance and coordination. Always remember: the goal is to support your health and your baby's growth, not to push your limits.

6.3. Setting Goals: Define What You Want to Achieve

When setting your prenatal workout goals, take a moment to define what you want to achieve. Is it building strength for labor? Maintaining cardiovascular health? Reducing pregnancy discomfort? Each goal may require different types of exercise, so it's vital to define them at the beginning.

6.4. Choosing the Right Exercises

Now comes the fun part - choosing your exercises! While you might need to adjust your routine as your baby grows and your body changes, here are some of the most beneficial exercises:

- Walking: Safe throughout all trimesters, walking is a low-impact exercise that boosts cardiovascular health, tones muscles, and can be done anywhere.

- Swimming: Water helps support your weight, reducing stress on your joints while you work on your stamina.

- Prenatal yoga: Yoga can increase your flexibility, improve your muscle-tone, and calm your mind.

- Prenatal Pilates: Pilates can help strengthen your core, improve posture, and alleviate backaches.

6.5. Creating Your Routine

When creating your routine, aim to include endurance training (like walking or swimming), strength training (like yoga or pilates), and relaxation techniques. Aim for at least 30 minutes of moderate-intensity exercise most days of the week, but remember, always listen to your body.

A sample week would look like:

- Monday: 30-minute brisk walk
- Tuesday: Prenatal yoga class
- Wednesday: Rest day
- Thursday: 30-minute swim
- Friday: Prenatal Pilates class
- Saturday: 30-minute brisk walk
- Sunday: Gentle yoga and relaxation

6.6. Listening to Your Body

Your body will always signal when you need to slow down. Look out for signs of overheating, like feeling dizzy or nauseated. Ensure you stay well-hydrated and avoid exercising in hot environments.

6.7. Conclusion

Remember, your health and that of your baby come first. So be gentle with yourself. The objective isn't to run a marathon but to stay active and prepare your body for the beautiful journey ahead. With the several benefits ranging from improved mood, enhanced strength, better sleep, and tailored birthing endurance, a carefully designed prenatal workout routine is a valuable asset for every expectant mother. Embrace this journey, knowing that with each step, each stroke, each pose, you're nurturing yourself and your growing baby. The practice of self-care in this period benefits you not just during pregnancy, but in motherhood and beyond. Enjoy every step of it!

Chapter 7. Delicious Recipes for a Nourished Pregnancy

Eating well is one of the most effective ways to provide for your growing baby's nutritional needs, and we're here to help! We have carefully curated mouth-watering, nutritious recipes that are perfect for every stage of pregnancy. From quick bites for curbing morning sickness to protein-packed main courses, here are plenty of options that won't disappoint.

7.1. The Importance of Nutrients in Pregnancy

A balanced diet is essential during pregnancy. Specific nutrients help foster your baby's growth while helping you maintain optimal health. Let's highlight the key nutritional components:

- Folate (also known as folic acid): Crucial for preventing neural tube defects.

- Iron: Aids in the development of your baby's bones and teeth.

- Vitamin D: Helps to absorb calcium effectively.

- Calcium: Necessary for the healthy development of bones and teeth.

- Protein: Essential for growth, particularly during the second and third trimester.

- Fiber: Helps maintain bowel health and prevent constipation, a common complaint during pregnancy.

7.2. Breakfast Recipes

Breakfast is the first feed your body gets after a night-long fast. It aids in replenishing the glucose levels needed to kick-start the day.

7.2.1. Nutty Granola with Greek Yogurt

Ingredients:

- 2 cups old fashioned oats
- 1 cup mixed unsalted nuts (e.g., almonds, walnuts)
- 1/2 cup mixed seeds (e.g., pumpkin, sunflower)
- 1 tablespoon honey
- 1 tablespoon coconut oil (melted)
- 1/2 cup dried fruits (e.g., raisins, apricots)
- 1 cup Greek yogurt

Steps:

1. Preheat the oven to 175°C (345°F).
2. Mix oats, nuts, and seeds in a large bowl. Stir in honey and coconut oil.
3. Spread the mixture on a baking sheet lined with parchment paper.
4. Bake for 20 minutes, stirring every 5 minutes to ensure even cooking.
5. Once golden brown, let it cool before mixing in the dried fruits.
6. Serve with Greek yogurt.

7.2.2. Avocado and Egg on Whole Grain Toast

Ingredients:

- 1 ripe avocado
- 2 eggs
- 2 slices whole grain bread
- Salt and black pepper to taste
- Chili flakes (optional)

Steps:

1. Cut the avocado in half and remove the pit. Scoop out the flesh and mash it with a fork.
2. Spread the mash onto toasted whole grain bread.
3. Cook the eggs to your preference and place on top of the avocado spread.
4. Season with salt, pepper, and optional chili flakes.

\n=== Lunch Recipes

Lunch will give you the necessary energy to keep you active through the afternoon. It also serves as an opportunity to add more fiber and essential nutrients to your diet.

7.2.3. Grilled Chicken Salad

Ingredients:

- 2 chicken breasts
- 4 cups mixed salad greens
- 1 cup cherry tomatoes (halved)
- 1 cucumber (sliced)

- 1 carrot (shredded)

- 1 tablespoon olive oil

- Salt and black pepper

Dressing:

- 3 tablespoons yogurt

- 1 tablespoon lemon juice

- 1 tablespoon honey

- Salt to taste

Steps:

1. Marinate the chicken in olive oil, salt, and black pepper for 15 minutes.

2. Grill until cooked (internal temperature should be 165°F). Slice the chicken.

3. Toss the salad greens, tomatoes, cucumber, and carrot together. Add sliced chicken on top.

4. Mix yogurt, lemon juice, honey, and salt to create the dressing, then drizzle over the salad.

7.2.4. Pumpkin and Lentil Soup

Ingredients:

- 2 cups diced pumpkin

- 1 cup red lentils

- 1 onion (chopped)

- 2 cloves garlic (minced)

- 1 tablespoon olive oil

- 4 cups vegetable stock

- Salt and pepper to taste

Steps:

1. Heat olive oil in a large pot. Add onions and garlic - sauté until translucent.

2. Add pumpkin and lentils to the pot, followed by the vegetable stock. Season with salt and pepper.

3. Bring to a boil, then reduce to simmer until the pumpkin and lentils are tender.

4. Blend until smooth, then season to taste.

7.3. Dinner Recipes

Serve up a nutrient-dense dinner that gives you a satiating end to the day while providing your body with overnight fuel.

7.3.1. Baked Salmon with Quinoa and Steamed Broccoli

Ingredients:

- 2 salmon fillets

- 1 cup quinoa

- 2 cups broccoli florets

- 2 tablespoons olive oil

- Salt and black pepper

- Lemon slices

Steps:

1. Preheat the oven to 180°C (350°F).

2. Place the salmon on a baking tray. Drizzle with olive oil and season with salt and pepper. Add lemon slices on top.

3. Bake for 20 minutes, or until the salmon flakes easily with a fork.

4. While the salmon bakes, prepare the quinoa according to package instructions.

5. Steam the broccoli until tender.

6. Serve salmon with a side of quinoa and steamed broccoli.

Remember, this is just a guideline. Everyone is unique and so are their nutritional needs. Always consult with your healthcare provider when altering your diet during pregnancy. Happy cooking!

Chapter 8. Listening to Your Body: Recognizing and Responding to Your Signals

From the moment you see the two lines on the pregnancy test stick, your body embarks on an extraordinary journey of transformation. Now, it is incumbent on you to listen and respond to its signals conscientiously. Pregnancy, though beautiful, is also a demanding time for your body—both physically and emotionally—and it's crucial to stay cognizant of, and responsive to, the changes occurring within you.

8.1. The Importance of Intuitive Listening

The essence of a fit pregnancy is intuitive listening to your body. It's about creating a harmonious balance between your physical needs, emotional demands, and the developmental requirements of your unborn little one. Unlike any fitness routine or diet program that follows a rigid structure, pregnancy is a uniquely personal experience defined by individual perception and bodily signals. Paying meticulous attention to these signs can help you navigate the changing tides of pregnancy smoothly.

You're not required to accomplish any Herculean feat of fitness or dietary excellence. You just need to do what's best for your body—and consequently, your baby. That means listening carefully to your body's signals, understanding what they mean, and taking responsive actions. Familiarizing yourself with common pregnancy symptoms and knowing when to seek professional advice can make the whole process less mystifying.

8.2. Physical Indicators – More Than Just Morning Sickness

In the early stages of pregnancy, your body undergoes immense hormonal changes leading to a variety of physical signals. Adapting and responding to these changes is crucial for building a healthy environment for your baby's growth.

Morning sickness, characterized by nausea and vomiting, is perhaps the most well-known sign. Though it tends to subside by the second trimester, each case differs. Not all expectant mothers experience these symptoms, and for some, it extends beyond the morning hours.

If you're suffering from severe morning sickness that prevents you from keeping down any food or fluids, it's important to contact your healthcare provider. It may be Hyperemesis Gravidarum, which requires medical intervention. Dehydration and weight loss are two prominent signals not to be overlooked.

Breasting changes is another common physical signaling during pregnancy. They can become larger, tender, and the veins more visible due to hormonal fluctuations. Accommodating for these changes, such as investing in a well-fitted maternity bra, provides necessary comfort and support.

Now, let's shift our focus to a comparatively less highlighted pregnancy signal—fatigue. It's normal as your body works overtime to support the developing baby, but excessive fatigue might indicate anemia. Regular check-ups enable early detection and management of this condition.

8.3. Emotional Indicators – Acknowledging Your Feelings

Equally vital as physical signals are your emotional cues. Hormonal changes can lead you to experience mood swings, anxiety, and sadness. It's crucial to understand that these fluctuations are normal and it's okay to seek support.

Talking about your feelings with your partner, friends, or a mental health professional can significantly alleviate stress. Furthermore, relaxation exercises can help maintain emotional equilibrium.

If feelings of sadness and anxiety persist, it's important to reach out to healthcare professionals without delay as it could be a sign of antenatal depression. Listening to these emotional signals in tandem with physical ones fosters a healthier pregnancy as mind and body closely interact and influence each other.

8.4. Key Takeaways

1. Understanding and responding to your body's signals are essential to a fit pregnancy.

2. Physical indicators like morning sickness, breast changes, and fatigue are all critical signs.

3. Listening to emotional cues and seeking support are vital for your mental wellbeing.

4. Regular consultations with your healthcare provider are crucial.

Ultimately, pregnancy is a unique journey for each woman. There's no universally perfect route, just the one that works best for you and your baby. It's about syncing with your body's rhythm, comprehending its cues, and doing what feels right. Keep in mind, taking care of your body is the first step in taking care of your baby.

Chapter 9. Safeguarding Against Common Pregnancy Complications

Pregnancy is an exciting time for many women, but it's also a period of immense change as your body makes room for and nurtures another human being. With these changes come a variety of possible complications. While the instances of these complications happening are not necessarily common, being prepared is crucial. Here, we'll dive into how you can safeguard against common pregnancy complications, by educating yourself about potential issues and discussing proven preventive measures.

9.1. Understanding the Basics

Before discussing how to prevent complications, it's important to understand what might come up during pregnancy. Issues ranging from gestational diabetes to hypertension, and preeclampsia to miscarriages can occur. By being informed, you can adopt habits that lower your risk and enhance the chances of a healthy and safe pregnancy.

9.2. Diet and Nutrition: Safeguarding Your Body

Watching what you eat isn't just for weight control—it's also for your overall health and the health of your unborn child. Pregnancy enhances the body's need for specific nutrients, including iron, calcium, and folate. Therefore, incorporating foods rich in these nutrients into your daily meals is crucial. Make sure your diet is diverse, primarily consisting of fresh fruits, vegetables, lean proteins, and whole grains. Supplementary vitamins and minerals may be recommended by your healthcare provider.

There's a strong link between diabetes and diet. Since gestational diabetes is a common complication, keeping a healthy diet can help prevent it. Foods high in fiber, low in sugars, and composed of complex carbohydrates are beneficial.

9.3. Staying Hydrated

Water plays a crucial part in nourishing your baby and sustaining a healthy pregnancy. It promotes amniotic fluid production, aids digestion, helps transport crucial nutrients to your baby and can prevent common problems such as constipation. As important as it is to hydrate, it's equally vital to limit intake of sugary drinks, which can spike blood sugar levels, potentially leading to gestational diabetes.

9.4. Regular Exercise

Regular physical activity can reinforce your body's ability to endure pregnancy's physical tolls. It helps your muscles remain robust and resilient, supports good cardiovascular health, and may lower the risk for gestational diabetes and preeclampsia. Exercise can help keep your weight within a healthy range, which is vital as excessive weight gain can lead to problems like gestational diabetes, preeclampsia, and increased risk for C-section delivery.

9.5. Importance of Prenatal Care

Regular prenatal check-ups are your primary defense against pregnancy complications. During these visits, your healthcare provider will check your and your baby's health. They may conduct ultrasounds, blood tests, and monitor your blood pressure. Through these regular check-ups, potential complications can be detected earlier and managed efficiently.

9.6. Managing Stress Levels

While occasional stress is part of life, chronic high stress can increase the risk of complications such as premature birth and low birth weight. It's important to recognize stress triggers and find healthy coping mechanisms.

9.7. Fostering a Smoke-Free and Substance-Free Environment

Avoiding smoking and alcohol during pregnancy is critical. Exposure to these can lead to congenital disabilities, premature birth, and other pregnancy complications.

Drawing on these aspects that safeguard against common pregnancy complications, you can better protect your health and your baby's while also ensuring a smoother journey through motherhood. It's about taking charge of your health, understanding potential risks, and doing your best to ensure your unborn child's wellbeing and your resilience as you prepare for one of life's most beautiful and rewarding challenges. Remember, every step you take towards a healthier pregnancy is a step towards a healthier start for your baby.

Chapter 10. Self Care Strategies: Maintaining Mental Well-being During Pregnancy

Expecting a baby is a life-altering event filled with joy, excitement, and anticipation. However, it can also bring stress, anxiety, and mood swings, taking a toll on your mental well-being. With hormonal changes and the physiological adjustments your body undergoes, it's entirely normal to experience a range of emotions. But with the right self-care strategies, you can maintain and even improve your mental wellness during this critical time in your life.

10.1. Understanding Emotional Changes and Stressors

Pregnancy is a journey with numerous physical, psychological, and emotional transitions. The hormonal changes in your body can contribute to mood swings and emotional instability. On top of this, various factors such as financial worries, body changes, and concerns about the baby's health can add stress. Acknowledging these emotions and stressors is the first step towards maintaining your mental well-being.

To help you navigate these changes, consider establishing open lines of communication with your partner, your health professionals, and your support network. It's essential not to bottle up feelings and seek interactions that provide comfort and understanding.

10.2. Creating a Support System

Building a strong support system is vital during pregnancy. Surrounding yourself with positive influences and people who genuinely care about you can provide a sense of security, belonging, and happiness. This support may come from your partner, family, friends, or even pregnancy support groups.

When you're pregnant, empathy and understanding from others can be immensely reassuring. Don't hesitate to share your concerns, feelings, and thoughts with these individuals. Creating a support system not only promotes your mental well-being but also offers an enriched environment for your growing baby.

10.3. Practising Mindfulness and Relaxation Techniques

Mindfulness is the practice of focusing on the present moment while calmly acknowledging and accepting one's feelings, thoughts, and bodily sensations. When you feel stressed or overwhelmed, try exercises such as deep breathing, progressive muscle relaxation, and guided imagery.

Meditation can also play a significant role in ensuring your mental wellness. There are numerous free resources and apps that offer guided meditations specifically designed for expectant mothers.

Another vital element to incorporate is regular physical exercise, which has proven benefits for managing stress and promoting a positive mood. Always consult with your doctor for appropriate exercises during each stage of your pregnancy.

10.4. Eating for Mental Health

Eating a balanced and nutritious diet plays an essential role in maintaining your mental well-being during pregnancy. Certain nutrients like omega-3 fatty acids, found in fish, walnuts and flaxseed, and B vitamins, found in leafy greens, beans, peas, and lentils, are known to help reduce symptoms of depression and anxiety.

Additionally, regularly eating small, balanced meals throughout the day can help maintain stable blood sugar levels, thereby preventing mood swings and irritability. Do not skip meals, and remember to hydrate well each day.

10.5. Taking Time Out for Yourself

Taking "me-time" can bring a wealth of benefits to your mental health. During this time, you could indulge in things that you love and enjoy – like reading, crafting, baking, or simply listening to your favorite music.

Another important aspect is rest and sleep. Pregnancy can take a toll on your energy levels, so it's crucial to listen to your body and get plenty of sleep.

10.6. Seeking Professional Help

Despite your best efforts, if you find your stress, anxiety, or mood swings overwhelming or persistent, it may be time to seek professional help. Therapists, counsellors, and psychiatrists are trained professionals who can provide you with effective strategies and treatments.

Always remember, caring for your mental health is not a luxury—it's a necessity. By tending to your emotional well-being, you are also creating a healthy and nurturing environment for your child. You're not alone in this journey, and it's okay to reach out for help.

Let this chapter be a guide to you, but remember, your journey is unique. Listen to your body, trust your instincts, and take care of both your physical and mental health. The road to motherhood is as beautiful as it is demanding, but with the right self-care strategies, you can enjoy a healthy and heartwarming pregnancy journey.

Chapter 11. Postpartum Recovery: Nutrition and Exercise for the New Mom

Proper nourishment and exercise play an integral role in helping a new mom regain her strength, rebuild her energy reserves, and lose pregnancy weight. When done right, they can also aid in combating postpartum depression and boosting overall mental well-being, therefore creating a healthier environment for nurturing the newborn. That said, postpartum recovery has to be gradual and well-monitored, ensuring that the new mom doesn't overstretch her body.

11.1. Nourishment: Refilling Your Body's Nutrient Reserves

During pregnancy, the body taps into its nutrient reserve to nourish both the mom and the baby. Once the baby is born, it is essential to replenish this reserve not only for the mom's health but also to fuel milk production for breastfeeding.

A balanced postpartum diet needs to be rich in:

- Proteins: Essential for tissue repair and regeneration. Include lean meat, eggs, dairy products, beans, lentils, and plant-based proteins in your diet.

- Iron: Prevent iron deficiency or anemia. Iron-rich foods include lean red meat, leafy green vegetables, legumes, and fortified cereals.

- Calcium: Critical for bone health. Dairy products, green leafy vegetables, and fortified plant-based milk are good sources.

- Fiber: Prevent constipation. Eat whole grains, fruits and

vegetables.

- Water: Essential for maintaining hydration and enhancing milk production. Aim to drink eight glasses of water a day or more.

NOTE While it is common to want to lose pregnancy weight quickly, it's vital to focus mainly on nourishing your body and not on rapid weight loss.

Breastfeeding moms need an extra 300-500 calories a day, which should come from nutrient-rich foods. Remember, the quality of the food you eat matters much more than the quantity.

11.2. Being Active: Gentle Exercise and Its Benefits

Getting active after childbirth may feel daunting, especially with the fatigue and body pain new moms often experience. However, light exercise promotes physical well-being and aids in recovery.

You can start with gentle exercises as soon as you feel comfortable and your doctor gives you the go ahead. Typically this might be a few days after a normal delivery or a little longer after a C-section.

Gentle exercises to consider:

- Walking: Start with short, leisurely walks and gradually increase the distance and pace. It will help improve circulation, supporting healing.

- Pelvic floor exercises: These strengthen muscles that support your uterus, bladder, and bowels. Strengthened pelvic muscles minimize the risk of incontinence.

- Gentle stretches: They ease body stiffness and improve flexibility, aiding in getting your body to adapt back post-pregnancy.

- Deep breathing exercises: Deep breaths can enhance oxygen circulation, aiding tissue repair, and relieving stress.

NOTE Always do warm-up exercises before starting and pace yourself to avoid any strain or discomfort. If you feel pain during an exercise, stop immediately.

11.3. Intensifying Your Workout: Safe Ways to Do It

Once you get comfortable with gentle exercises and your body heals sufficiently (usually around 6-8 weeks, but this varies from person to person), you can try more intensive workouts. Always consult with your healthcare provider before intensifying your workouts.

Here are a few more challenging workouts to consider:

- Yoga and Pilates: These help in toning your body and strengthening the core.

- Aerobic exercises: Activities like swimming, jogging, or cycling boost heart health and promote weight loss.

- Strength-training exercises: Using light weights can aid in toning muscles and enhancing overall stamina.

Striking the right balance between nutrition and exercise will ensure a smoother recovery process and a more energized you, who can fully enjoy the incredible journey of motherhood. So be kind to your body, prioritize your needs, and have patience with the process. Remember, you've just accomplished the miracle of life!

11.4. Postpartum Depression: Recognizing the Signs and Getting Help

One vital aspect of postpartum recovery often overlooked is emotional wellbeing. Up to 80% of new moms experience a form of postpartum mood disorder, from mild baby blues to the more serious postpartum depression (PPD).

Common symptoms of PPD include:

- Constant sadness or tearfulness

- Overwhelming fatigue or insomnia

- Feelings of worthlessness or guilt

- Lack of interest or joy in life

- Withdrawal from family and friends

If you recognize these signs in yourself, it's essential to seek help. Talk to a healthcare provider who can guide you to the right treatment or support group. You are not alone, and there's assistance available. Just as you nourish your body, feed your emotional health too - for your sake and your baby's.

Remember, motherhood is a journey. It doesn't have to be perfect; it simply has to be 'you'. So take one day at a time, breathe, and celebrate the little victories. Your strength is the best legacy you can leave for your child. Trust your instincts, love yourself, and be the best version of you because, ultimately, a happy mom means a happy baby.

www.ingramcontent.com/pod-product-compliance
Lightning Source LLC
Chambersburg PA
CBHW071015260726
48661CB00007B/2964